PETS MAKE PEOPLE BETTER

The Health Benefits of Pet Companionship

Kevin B DiBacco

author, except as permitted by U.S. copyright law.
Published by Chelsea House Press Inc.

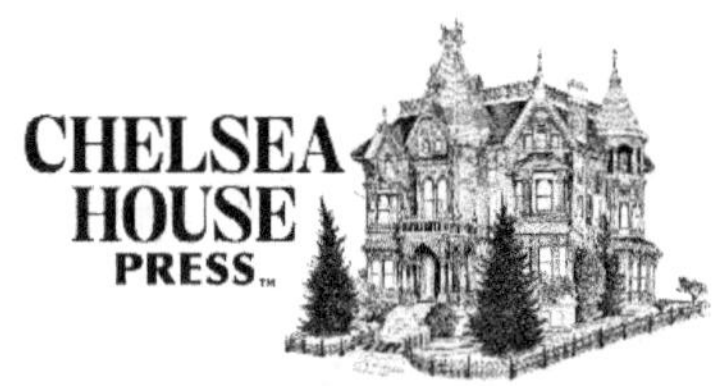

1

without the prior written permission of the copyright holder. The author has tried to present information that is as correct and concrete as possible. The author is not a medical doctor and does not write in any medical capacity. All medical decisions should be made under the guidance and care of your primary physician. The author will not be held liable for any injury or loss that is incurred to the reader through the application of any of the information here contained in this book. The author makes it clear that the medical field is fast evolving with newer studies being done continuously, therefore the information in this book is only a researched collaboration of accurate information at the time of writing. With the ever-changing nature of the subjects included, the author hopes that the reader will be able to appreciate the content that has been covered in this book. While all attempts have been made to verify each piece of information provided in this publication, the author assumes no responsibility for any error, omission, or contrary interpretation of the subject matter present in this book. Please note that any help or advice given hereof is not a substitution for licensed medical advice. The reader accepts responsibility in the use of any information and takes advice given in this book at their own risk. If the reader is under medication supervision or has had complications with health-related risks, consult your primary care physician as soon as possible before taking any advice given in this book.

"The information and advice contained in this book are based upon the research and the personal and professional experiences of the author. They are not intended as a substitute for consulting with a healthcare professional. The publisher and author are not responsible for any adverse effects or consequences resulting from the use of any of the suggestions, preparations, or procedures discussed in this book. All matters pertaining to your physical health should be supervised by a healthcare professional."

About the Author

Kevin understands adversity and the temptation to quit better than most. His life has been a testament to the power of perseverance despite severe hardship. Now, he shares his story and tools to inspire others to get off the mat when knocked down by life.

Kevin's health struggles began early, needing major surgery at just 16 years old. In his 20s and 30s, he endured 6 knee operations, 2 back surgeries, including spinal fusion, 2 hip replacements, and treatment for an aggressive brain tumor. Enduring over 10 major medical procedures would be enough to make anyone want to give up. Even as he was writing this, Kevin was struck by Covid-19. As if that wasn't another setback, Kevin developed Pneumonia and spent the spring of 2022 and the summer of 2023 having to get daily nebulizer treatments. Once again, his theories were put to the test. Once again, they worked!

But Kevin refused to see himself as a victim of circumstance. Through each diagnosis and rehabilitation, he consciously worked to reframe adversity as an opportunity for growth. Instead of sadly ruminating on limitations, he focused positively on each small win - standing, walking, and climbing stairs - during recovery. He visualized himself healed and happy against all odds.

Kevin leaned on his deep faith and the support of loved ones during the darkest times. When fear or hopelessness crept in, he prayed for the strength to take the next step forward. He turned to uplifting books and sayings for encouragement. Slowly but surely, he reclaimed his active lifestyle step by step.

Through his journey, Kevin realized firsthand the power of mindset to decide one's life experience. He discovered that he could transform his outer reality by controlling his inner world - his thoughts, beliefs, and visualizations. Now, he hopes to share these lessons with others facing major life challenges.

Kevin's book recounts his medical battles, along with the techniques he used to stay grounded in positivity. He provides exercises to overcome negative self-talk, face fears, and visualize desired outcomes. Kevin believes we can all learn to reframe difficulties as growth opportunities. Wherever we feel like quitting, he urges us to proclaim, "I will keep going!"

Kevin's dramatic story provides living proof that, no matter what knocks us down, we can choose to get back up. We all have access to inner reserves of strength to endure the unendurable. Kevin hopes his book will inspire others to fight major life battles to find their power to keep progressing. By committing to personal growth, we can overcome any obstacle, including those within our own minds.

Chapter 1: The Healing Power of Pets

The Connection Between Pets and Health

Subchapter: The Connection Between Pets and Health

Welcome to the enlightening subchapter of "Pets Make Better People: Unlocking the Health Benefits of Pet Companionship." Whether you are a lifelong pet lover or someone considering bringing a furry friend into your life, this chapter aims to shed light on the profound connection between pets and health. Brace yourselves for an exploration of how life truly becomes better when you have pets!

The Healing Power of Pets:

Pets, in all their adorable and unconditional love, have a remarkable impact on our mental well-being. Numerous studies have shown that pet companionship can alleviate symptoms of anxiety, depression, and loneliness. The simple act of petting a dog or stroking a cat can release oxytocin, a hormone responsible for reducing stress and promoting feelings of happiness. Pets offer a soothing presence, lending a listening ear without judgment, and providing comfort during challenging times.

Boosting Overall Happiness:

The presence of pets in our lives can significantly enhance our overall happiness. They bring joy and laughter, infuse our routines with purpose, and motivate us to stay active and engaged. Pets provide a sense of belonging and companionship, helping us combat feelings of isolation. Whether it's a wagging tail, a purr, or a chirp, their unique ways of communicating fill our lives with immense love and joy.

Reducing Stress and Anxiety:

Stress and anxiety have become all too common in our lives. However, studies have revealed that petting or interacting with animals can lower blood pressure, reduce heart rate, and diminish stress hormones. Pets create a calming environment, promoting a sense of tranquility and mindfulness. They offer a distraction from daily worries, allowing us to focus on the present moment and find solace in their company.

Supporting Emotional Well-being:

Pets also play a crucial role in supporting our emotional well-being. They act as empathetic companions, sensing our moods and offering unconditional love and support. For individuals struggling with health issues, pets can provide a sense of purpose, responsibility, and routine. They offer a source of emotional stability and help us develop empathy and compassion.

Conclusion:

Overall, the connection between pets and health is a profound and transformative one. Pets have an incredible ability to heal, bring happiness, reduce stress, and support our emotional well-being. Whether it's a wagging tail, a gentle purr, or a playful chirp, pets remind us of that life truly is better when we have them by our side. So, embrace the wonders of pet companionship and unlock the countless health benefits that come with it.

The History of Pet Therapy

Humans have always had a special bond with animals, and throughout history, this bond has been recognized and harnessed for its therapeutic benefits. The concept of pet therapy, also known as animal-assisted therapy, is not a recent phenomenon. In fact, its roots can be traced back to ancient civilizations.

In Ancient Egypt, animals, particularly cats, were revered for their healing abilities. Cats were believed to have mystical powers that could ward off evil spirits and bring comfort to those in need. Similarly, in Ancient

Greece, dogs were used as therapy animals to provide emotional support and companionship to individuals with health conditions.

The modern concept of pet therapy, as we know it today, gained traction in the 18th century. It was during this time that the medical community began to recognize the positive impact animals could have on human well-being. In the early 1790s, Quaker retreats in England started incorporating animals into their treatment plans, finding that patients responded positively to the presence of animals, experiencing reduced anxiety and improved mood.

During World War II, pet therapy gained further recognition when it was discovered that dogs could provide immense comfort and emotional support to wounded soldiers. The famous war dog, Smoky, became a symbol of hope and healing for soldiers as she went with them on dangerous missions and provided much-needed companionship during their recovery.

In the 1960s, pet therapy started to be formally incorporated into healthcare settings. The renowned child psychiatrist, Dr. Boris Levinson, discovered that his dog, Jingles, had a profound effect on his young patients. Jingles helped children open, express their emotions, and build trust, leading to significant breakthroughs in therapy sessions. This groundbreaking work paved the way for the integration of pet therapy into various medical and health settings.

Today, pet therapy is widely recognized for its ability to improve health and overall well-being. Research has shown that interacting with animals can lower blood pressure, reduce stress and anxiety, alleviate symptoms of depression, and improve social interactions. It is now a common practice in hospitals, nursing homes, schools, and rehabilitation centers, where trained therapy animals work alongside healthcare professionals to provide comfort, support, and companionship to patients and individuals in need.

As humans, we have always known that life is better when we have pets. The history of pet therapy is a testament to the profound impact animals can have on our health. Whether it's the ancient Egyptians recognizing the healing powers of cats or modern-day hospitals incorporating therapy dogs into their treatment plans, the bond between humans and animals continues to unlock the health benefits of pet companionship.

The Rise of Pet Companionship

Pets have always held a special place in our hearts, but recently, their significance in our lives has reached new heights. The bond between humans and animals has evolved into a companionship that goes beyond mere ownership. Today, pets are not just pets; they are cherished members of our families, bringing immeasurable joy, comfort, and love into our lives. This subchapter explores the rise of pet companionship and the reasons why life is undeniably better when you have pets.

One of the most compelling reasons for the surge in pet companionship is the growing awareness of the health benefits they offer. Scientific research has shown that interacting with pets can have a profound positive impact on our emotional well-being. The unconditional love and unwavering loyalty pets provide can alleviate feelings of loneliness, reduce stress, and even help combat depression and anxiety. In a world where stress and health issues are on the rise, pets have become a source of solace, offering a listening ear and a comforting presence.

Likewise, pets have a remarkable ability to bring people together. They act as social catalysts, breaking down barriers and fostering connections among individuals. Whether it's at a dog park or a neighborhood gathering, pets serve as conversation starters, helping us forge new friendships and strengthen existing ones. Their presence encourages us to engage with others, promoting social interaction and reducing feelings of isolation.

Added to their emotional benefits, pets also contribute to our physical well-being. Owning a pet often entails regular exercise, whether it's taking them for walks, playing fetch, or engaging in other activities. This increased physical activity improves our fitness levels and boosts our overall health. Pets can also provide a sense of purpose and responsibility, as their care and well-being become our top priority.

Additionally, pets offer a unique form of therapy, particularly for children and the elderly. Studies have shown that interaction with animals can enhance cognitive and social development in children, while also providing a sense of routine and stability. For the elderly, pets can alleviate feelings of loneliness and provide companionship during challenging times.

The rise of pet companionship is a testament to the profound impact animals have on our lives. They bring us joy, comfort, and love, while also improving our mental and physical well-being. Whether you're a dog lover, a cat person, or have a penchant for more exotic animals, the benefits of pet companionship are universal. Life is indeed better when you have pets, as they enrich our lives in countless ways, reminding us of the beauty and simplicity of unconditional love.

Chapter 2: Understanding Pet Therapy

Defining Pet Therapy

Pets have always been an integral part of human lives, bringing joy, companionship, and unconditional love. However, their impact goes far beyond just being great companions. Lately, there has been a growing recognition of the health benefits that pets can provide. This subchapter aims to delve into the concept of pet therapy, exploring its definition and the positive effects it can have on our overall well-being.

Pet therapy, also known as animal-assisted therapy or AAT, is a therapeutic intervention that involves the use of animals to improve human health and well-being. It is a structured and goal-oriented approach that uses the innate connection between humans and animals to achieve specific therapeutic outcomes. Pet therapy is not limited to a particular age group or health condition; it can be beneficial for all humans.

The primary goal of pet therapy is to enhance the quality of life and promote healing by providing emotional support, reducing stress, and improving social interaction. Interacting with animals, such as dogs, cats, horses, or even smaller pets like rabbits or guinea pigs, has been proven to release endorphins, reduce anxiety, and lower blood pressure. These physiological changes contribute to a sense of calmness and overall well-being.

As well as the physical benefits, pet therapy also offers psychological advantages. The presence of animals can provide comfort and emotional support to individuals struggling with depression, anxiety, or loneliness. Pets have a unique ability to provide unconditional love and acceptance, creating a safe space for individuals to express their emotions without fear of judgment.

Pet therapy has shown remarkable results in various settings, including hospitals, nursing homes, schools, and rehabilitation centers. It has been effective in helping children with autism elevate their social skills, elderly individuals with dementia regain cognitive abilities, and patients with health disorders experience a reduction in symptoms.

Pet therapy has become increasingly recognized as a valuable tool in promoting health and well-being. It offers a comprehensive approach to healing, addressing emotional, psychological, and physical aspects of human health. Whether you are struggling with a health condition or simply looking to enhance your overall wellness, pet therapy can be a transformative experience.

In the following chapters, we will explore the different approaches to pet therapy, the specific benefits it offers, and how you can incorporate pets into your life to unlock their health benefits. Remember, life is better when you have pets!

Different Approaches to Pet Therapy

Pets have long been recognized for their ability to bring joy, comfort, and companionship to our lives. However, their impact on our health goes far beyond the surface of happiness. Pet therapy, also known as animal-assisted therapy, is a specialized form of treatment that uses the unique bond between humans and animals to improve overall well-being. In this subchapter, we will explore different approaches to pet therapy, highlighting the various ways in which pets can positively affect our health.

One approach to pet therapy is known as "Animal-Assisted Activities" (AAA). This approach involves bringing animals, such as dogs or cats, into various settings, such as hospitals, nursing homes, or schools, to provide comfort and companionship to individuals in need. The presence of these animals can help reduce stress, anxiety, and feelings of loneliness, while also promoting social interaction and improving overall mood.

Another approach is "Animal-Assisted Therapy" (AAT), which involves working with a trained therapy animal under the guidance of a healthcare professional. AAT sessions are tailored to meet specific therapeutic goals, such as improving communication skills, increasing self-esteem, or reducing symptoms of post-traumatic stress disorder. These sessions can take place in a clinical setting or even at home, depending on the individual's needs.

Equine-assisted therapy is a unique approach that involves interactions with horses. Horses have a remarkable ability to mirror human emotions and provide immediate feedback. Through activities such as grooming, riding, or simply being in their presence, individuals can develop trust, improve emotional regulation, and enhance their overall sense of well-being.

For those who may not have access to animals or have allergies, virtual pet therapy is an emerging approach that uses technology to provide the benefits of pet companionship. Virtual pet therapy involves interacting with realistic virtual pets through apps or virtual reality. These digital companions can provide comfort, relaxation, and a sense of responsibility without the need for physical presence.

Overall, these different approaches to pet therapy prove the versatility and effectiveness of incorporating pets into our lives for health benefits. Whether it's through Animal-Assisted Activities, Animal-Assisted Therapy, equine-assisted therapy, or even virtual pet therapy, pets have the power to uplift and improve our mental well-being. So, why not embrace the idea that "Life is better when you have pets!" and explore the incredible world of pet therapy for yourself?

The Role of Animals in Therapy

In today's fast-paced and stressful world, finding effective ways to improve health and well-being has become increasingly important. Fortunately, one powerful solution lies right at our fingertips, the companionship of animals. This subchapter explores the astounding role animals play in therapy and how they can significantly enhance our overall wellness.

The Healing Power of Animal Companionship:

Animals have an innate ability to provide unconditional love, support, and comfort to humans. Numerous studies have shown that spending time with animals can lower blood pressure, reduce anxiety and stress levels, and even alleviate symptoms of depression. As a result, therapists and medical professionals have started incorporating animal-assisted therapy into their treatment plans.

Animal-Assisted Therapy:

Animal-assisted therapy involves the use of trained animals to enhance a person's physical, emotional, cognitive, and social well-being. Dogs, cats, horses, and even exotic animals like dolphins and birds are utilized in various therapeutic settings. The presence of these animals can create a calming and safe environment, allowing individuals to open and express their emotions more freely.

Benefits of Animal-Assisted Therapy:

Animal-assisted therapy has proven to be beneficial for individuals of all ages and backgrounds. For children with autism, animals can help improve social interactions and communication skills. In elderly care facilities, animals provide companionship and reduce feelings of loneliness and isolation. Veterans suffering from post-traumatic stress disorder (PTSD) often find solace and relief through interacting with therapy animals. The positive impact of animals on health is truly remarkable.

Emotional Support Animals:

Beyond formal therapy settings, many individuals receive help from having emotional support animals (ESAs). ESAs provide comfort, companionship, and emotional support to individuals experiencing various health conditions. These animals are regularly prescribed by health professionals to help alleviate symptoms of anxiety, depression, and PTSD. The presence of an ESA can provide a sense of purpose, routine, and unconditional love, greatly improving the overall quality of life for their human companions.

Conclusion:

In a world where stress and health issues are prevalent, animals offer a unique and valuable form of therapy. Their ability to provide unconditional love, support, and companionship is truly remarkable. Animal-assisted therapy and emotional support animals have proven to be powerful tools in promoting mental well-being and enhancing the overall quality of life. So, whether you're struggling with health issues or simply seeking a boost in your well-being, consider opening your heart and home to the incredible healing power of animals. Remember, life is better when you have pets!

Chapter 3: The Emotional Benefits of Pet Companionship

Reducing Stress and Anxiety

Life is better when you have pets! These furry companions not only bring joy and love into our lives but also offer unbelievable health benefits. In this subchapter, we will explore how pets can help reduce stress and anxiety and provide practical tips for incorporating them into your wellness routine.

Pets, whether they are dogs, cats, or even smaller critters like rabbits or birds, have an uncanny ability to sense our emotions. They are natural stress relievers and can help us cope with the challenges of daily life. Studies have shown that interacting with pets can lower blood pressure, release calming hormones, and reduce anxiety levels. The simple act of petting or cuddling with a pet can promote relaxation and provide a sense of comfort.

Pets also encourage us to stay active and engage in physical activities. Regular exercise is a proven stress buster, and having a pet companion can motivate us to get moving. Whether it's taking your dog for a walk, playing fetch in the park, or even taking part in agility training, these activities help your pet's health and uplift your mood and reduce stress.

Plus, pets offer companionship and unconditional love, which can be particularly helpful during times of loneliness or isolation. They provide a sense of purpose and responsibility, giving us something to care for and nurture. The bond formed with a pet can bring immense emotional support, reducing feelings of anxiety and depression.

To make the most of the health benefits of pet companionship, it's essential to incorporate them into your daily routine. Here are a few tips to get started:

1. Spend quality time with your pet: Dedicate specific moments during the day to play, cuddle, or groom your furry friend. This interaction will strengthen your bond and help you relax.

2. Create a pet-friendly environment: Ensure your home is safe and comfortable for your pet. Providing them with cozy bedding, toys, and a designated space will make them feel secure and content.

3. Practice mindfulness with your pet: Engage in activities such as meditation or deep breathing exercises while enjoying your pet's presence. This will help you stay present, reduce stress, and strengthen your connection.

4. Join pet-related communities: Connect with other pet owners through social media groups or local clubs. Sharing experiences, tips, and stories can enhance your pet companionship journey and provide a support network.

In general, it can be said that having a pet in your life can significantly contribute to reducing stress and anxiety. By embracing the love and companionship they offer, you can unlock the health benefits that come with pet ownership. Incorporate these furry friends into your wellness routine and experience the joy and calm they bring to your life. Remember, life is better when you have pets!

Enhancing Mood and Happiness

Life is better when you have pets! There's no denying the joy and happiness that our furry friends bring into our lives. But did you know that pet companionship goes beyond just being adorable and cuddly? In this subchapter, we will explore the incredible health benefits that come with having a pet, and how they can enhance your mood and overall happiness.

Pets have a unique ability to bring a smile to our faces, even on the gloomiest of days. Whether it's the wagging tail of a dog or the purring of a cat, their presence alone can instantly lift our spirits. But there's more to it than just their cute antics. Studies have shown that spending time with a pet can release endorphins, also known as the "feel-good" hormones, in our brains. These endorphins help reduce stress, anxiety, and depression, leaving us feeling happier and more content.

One of the ways pets enhance our mood is through their unconditional love and companionship. They provide us with a sense of belonging and purpose, which can be especially valuable during challenging times. Having a pet to care for gives us a sense of responsibility and routine, helping us stay grounded and focused. Additionally, pets offer a listening ear without judgment, allowing us to express our thoughts and emotions freely, which can be incredibly therapeutic.

Pets also encourage us to be more active and social. Taking your dog for a walk or playing with your cat provides physical exercise and boosts our mood by increasing serotonin and dopamine levels. As well, pets can be excellent icebreakers, helping us connect with other pet owners and form new friendships. These social interactions are vital for our mental well-being, as they combat feelings of loneliness and isolation.

The positive impact of pets on our health extends beyond just the emotional realm. Studies have proven that pet owners have lower blood pressure and cholesterol levels, reduced risk of heart disease, and improved immune function. The simple act of petting a dog or cat can trigger the release of oxytocin, a hormone associated with bonding and relaxation, leading to a calmer and more peaceful state of mind.

To review, there's no doubt that having a pet can significantly enhance our mood and overall happiness. They provide us with unwavering love, companionship, and a multitude of health benefits. So, if you're looking for a natural and effective way to boost your well-being, consider welcoming a pet into your life. The joy and happiness they bring are truly unparalleled, and life is undeniably better with them by our side.

Building Emotional Resilience

It is essential to develop emotional resilience to navigate through life's challenges. One powerful tool that can help us with this journey is the companionship of pets. Whether you are a dog lover, a cat enthusiast, or prefer the company of another furry friend, the presence of pets can significantly contribute to building emotional resilience.

Pets have an innate ability to connect with us on a deep emotional level. They provide unwavering support, unconditional love, and a non-judgmental presence. This relationship can be a source of comfort, solace, and stability when we face adversity or difficult times. Research has shown that interacting with pet's releases oxytocin, often referred to as the "love hormone," which helps reduce stress, anxiety, and promotes emotional well-being.

One of the keyways pets aid in building emotional resilience is by teaching us valuable life skills. They teach us patience, as we learn to understand their needs and communicate effectively. They also teach us responsibility, as we become accountable for their well-being. Additionally, pets can help us develop empathy and compassion, as we learn to recognize and respond to their emotions.

The fact is that the presence of pets encourages us to engage in physical activity and support a healthy lifestyle. Regular walks, playtime, and outdoor activities with pets help their well-being and boost our physical and physical health. Exercise releases endorphins, which can elevate our mood, reduce stress, and increase our overall resilience.

Pets also provide us with a sense of purpose and belonging. They become part of our family, and their presence reminds us that we are needed and loved. This feeling of belongingness fosters a sense of security and stability, which is crucial in building emotional resilience.

Overall, pets have a remarkable influence on our emotional well-being and can play a crucial role in building emotional resilience. Their unconditional love, ability to teach us important life skills, and the joy they bring into our lives can help us navigate through life's challenges with greater strength and resilience. So, whether you already have a beloved pet or are considering adopting one, remember that life is indeed better when you have pets! Embrace their companionship, cherish their love, and allow them to support you in building emotional resilience.

Chapter 4: The Health Benefits of Pet Companionship

Alleviating Symptoms of Depression

Depression affects millions of people worldwide, casting a dark shadow over their lives and making each day a struggle. In the pursuit of finding effective methods to alleviate the symptoms of depression, researchers have stumbled upon an unexpected yet powerful solution – the companionship of pets. In this subchapter, we will explore how pets can play a transformative role in combating depression and bringing joy back into our lives.

Depression often leads to feelings of isolation and loneliness, making it difficult for individuals to connect with others. However, the presence of a pet can break down those barriers and provide a constant source of unconditional love and support. Pets, whether they are dogs, cats, or even smaller critters, have an innate ability to sense our emotions and provide comfort in times of distress. The simple act of stroking a pet's fur or hearing their gentle purring can evoke a sense of calm and tranquility, easing the burden of depression.

Besides emotional support, pets also encourage physical activity and social interaction, both of which are crucial for combating depression. Dogs need regular walks and playtime, which not only helps their well-being but also gives an opportunity for their owners to engage in physical exercise. Regular exercise releases endorphins, the body's natural mood-enhancing chemicals, thereby reducing the symptoms of depression and improving overall mental well-being.

Pets also offer a sense of purpose and responsibility, which can be invaluable for individuals struggling with depression. Taking care of a pet, ensuring they are well-fed, groomed, and loved, gives individuals a reason to get out of bed in the morning and offers a sense of accomplishment. This responsibility can provide a much-needed distraction from negative thoughts and help individuals regain a sense of control over their lives.

Additionally, the presence of pets has been shown to decrease stress levels and lower blood pressure, both of which are associated with depression. The act of petting a dog or cat has a calming effect, reducing anxiety and promoting a sense of relaxation. These physical benefits, combined with the emotional support pets provide, contribute to an overall improvement in health.

To summarize, pets have the remarkable ability to alleviate symptoms of depression and enhance our overall well-being. Their unwavering companionship, ability to reduce stress, encourage physical activity, and provide a sense of purpose can make a world of difference for individuals battling depression. By recognizing the health benefits of pet companionship, we can unlock a powerful tool in our journey towards happiness and personal fulfillment. So, let us embrace the message of this book: life is better when you have pets!

Easing Loneliness and Isolation

Pets have long been recognized as loyal companions and sources of comfort, but their impact on health goes far beyond simple companionship. In a world where loneliness and isolation are becoming increasingly prevalent, pets offer a unique and invaluable solution. This subchapter explores the profound ways in which pets can ease feelings of loneliness and isolation, offering a lifeline of connection and support to people from all occupations.

Loneliness can be a debilitating experience, affecting people of all ages and backgrounds. Yet, when we bring a pet into our lives, we open the door to a constant and unwavering source of companionship. Whether it's a dog enthusiastically wagging its tail or a cat purring contentedly on our lap, pets provide a tangible presence that can help alleviate feelings of emptiness and isolation. They offer a listening ear without judgment, and their unwavering presence can provide a sense of security and comfort, even during the darkest times.

Isolation, on the other hand, often stems from a lack of social connection or a feeling of being misunderstood. Pets bridge this gap effortlessly. They offer a shared language that transcends words, allowing us to communicate and form in-depth bonds based on love and understanding. Whether it's a walk in the park with a canine companion or a quiet evening spent cuddling with a feline friend, pets give us a sense of belonging and acceptance that can be difficult to find elsewhere.

Pets have shown remarkable abilities to detect and respond to emotional distress. They are attuned to our moods, offering a comforting presence when we are feeling down and celebrating with us during moments of joy. Their intuitive nature and ability to provide unconditional love make them invaluable allies in the battle against loneliness and isolation.

It is not surprising then that studies have consistently shown the positive impact of pet companionship on health. From reducing symptoms of anxiety and depression to improving overall well-being, pets have the power to transform lives. They encourage social interactions, provide a sense of purpose, and offer a daily dose of laughter and joy.

Life can often feel overwhelming, having a pet by your side can be a lifeline. So, whether you are young or old, single or surrounded by a bustling family, consider opening your heart and home to a furry friend. Embrace the incredible power of pet companionship and unlock a world where loneliness and isolation become distant memories. Life is better when you have pets!

Supporting Trauma Recovery

Trauma can have long-lasting effects on an individual's mental and emotional well-being. The journey towards healing and recovery can be challenging and typically requires a comprehensive approach. One powerful tool that has gained recognition for its positive impact on trauma recovery is pet companionship. The unwavering love, support, and companionship that pets provide can be instrumental in helping individuals navigate the path to healing.

Pets offer a unique form of support that is unmatched by any other intervention. Their presence alone can create a sense of safety and security, which is crucial for trauma survivors who may struggle with feelings of vulnerability. Whether it's a loyal dog, a calming cat, or a friendly rabbit, the unconditional love and non-judgmental nature of pets creates a safe space where survivors can begin to rebuild trust and explore their emotions.

The therapeutic benefits of pets extend beyond emotional support. Interacting with animals has been shown to reduce anxiety, lower blood pressure, and release endorphins, which are natural mood boosters. These physiological responses help trauma survivors manage their symptoms and promote a sense of overall well-being. Pets provide a distraction from intrusive thoughts and offer a positive focus for survivors, allowing them to experience moments of joy and connection.

In addition to the emotional and physiological benefits, pets can also help the development of important coping skills. Caring for a pet requires responsibility, routine, and structure, elements that can be particularly beneficial for individuals struggling with the aftermath of trauma. The process of feeding, grooming, and exercising a pet encourages survivors to show healthy habits, create a sense of purpose, and regain a sense of control over their lives.

It is essential to note that while pets can be incredibly supportive, they are not a substitute for professional help. Trauma survivors should seek therapy and counseling to address their underlying issues. However, incorporating pet companionship into the recovery process can enhance therapy outcomes and provide an added layer of support.

As a result, pets have a remarkable ability to support trauma recovery. Their unwavering love, non-judgmental nature, and therapeutic benefits make them invaluable companions on the healing journey. By providing a sense of safety, promoting emotional well-being, and facilitating the development of coping skills, pets can significantly contribute to a survivor's recovery process. Whether it's a dog, cat, rabbit, or any other animal, the presence of a pet can make a profound difference in an individual's life. As we navigate the challenges of trauma recovery, let us remember that life is indeed better when we have pets!

Chapter 5: Pet Therapy in Specific Populations

Pet Therapy for Children and Adolescents

In our fast-paced and technology-driven society, the health of children and adolescents is becoming an increasing concern. The pressures of school, social interactions, and the constant exposure to screens can have a detrimental impact on their well-being. However, there is a remarkable solution that can significantly improve their health and overall happiness with pet therapy. This subchapter explores the incredible benefits of pet therapy specifically for children and adolescents and why having pets in their lives can be a significant change.

Benefits of Pet Therapy:

Pets have an extraordinary ability to connect with humans on a deep emotional level, and this bond is particularly powerful for children and adolescents. Pet therapy offers many benefits that contribute to their health and overall well-being.

1. Emotional Support:

Pets provide unconditional love and support, creating a safe and non-judgmental environment for children and adolescents. They can be a source of comfort during times of stress, anxiety, or sadness, helping kids navigate their emotions with ease.

2. Social and Communication Skills:

Having a pet encourages social interaction, as children often engage in conversations about their furry friends with their peers. This interaction helps them develop communication and social skills, boosting their confidence and self-esteem.

3. Responsibility and Empathy:

Taking care of a pet instills a sense of responsibility in children and adolescents. They learn the importance of feeding, grooming, and providing affection to their furry companions. This responsibility fosters empathy, teaching them to consider the needs and feelings of others.

4. Stress Reduction:

Interacting with pets has a calming effect on children and adolescents, reducing stress levels and promoting relaxation. Spending time with animals has been proven to lower blood pressure and release endorphins, enhancing their overall mental well-being.

5. Health Support:

Pets can be beneficial for children and adolescents struggling with health issues such as depression or anxiety. The presence of a loving companion can alleviate symptoms, improve mood, and provide a sense of purpose and stability.

Today children and adolescents are facing increasing health challenges, pet therapy provides a remarkable solution. The benefits of having pets in their lives are undeniable, offering emotional support, fostering social skills, promoting responsibility and empathy, reducing stress, and supporting their health. Integrating pet therapy into their lives can pave the way for happier, healthier, and more fulfilling childhoods and adolescences. So, let's embrace the magic of pet companionship and unlock the health benefits it brings to our young ones. After all, life is undeniably better when you have pets!

Pet Therapy for Older Adults

As we age, keeping good mental and emotional well-being becomes increasingly important. One effective and enjoyable way to achieve this is through pet therapy. In this subchapter, we will explore the incredible benefits that pets can provide for older adults. Whether you are a senior citizen, a family member, or a caregiver, understanding how pet companionship can improve the quality of life for older adults is essential.

The Power of Pet Companionship:

Pets offer unconditional love, companionship, and a sense of purpose. For older adults, who may experience feelings of loneliness or isolation, having a pet can significantly enhance their emotional well-being. The presence of a furry friend can provide comfort, reduce stress, and alleviate symptoms of anxiety and depression.

Physical and Cognitive Benefits:

Pet therapy is not just about emotional support; it also brings many physical and cognitive advantages for older adults. Regular interaction with pets can encourage physical activity, such as walking or playing, resulting in improved cardiovascular health and increased mobility. Additionally, engaging with a pet can stimulate cognitive functions, improve memory, and enhance overall mental agility.

Reducing Health Risks:

Studies have shown that pet ownership can lead to a lower risk of certain health issues common in older adults. Having a pet can help regulate blood pressure, reduce the risk of heart disease, and even decrease the likelihood of falls. The routine and responsibility of caring for a pet also encourage healthier habits, such as regular exercise and supporting a consistent daily routine.

Social Connection and Increased Happiness:

Pets are natural conversation starters and can facilitate social interactions for older adults. Whether it's meeting fellow pet owners during walks or sharing stories about their furry companions, pets serve as a common ground for building friendships and fostering a sense of community. It is a fact, the presence of a pet often brings joy, laughter, and a renewed sense of purpose, which can have a profound impact on an older adult's overall happiness and mental well-being.

Incorporating pet therapy into the lives of older adults can unlock a multitude of health benefits. Pets provide companionship, reduce feelings of loneliness, and offer physical and cognitive stimulation. They can also help reduce health risks and increase social connections, ultimately leading to a happier and healthier life. Whether you are an older adult or someone caring for a senior, remember that life is indeed better when you have pets!

Pet Therapy in Hospital Settings Subchapter: Pet Therapy in Hospital Settings

In the stressful environment of a hospital, finding ways to promote healing and well-being is crucial. One unconventional yet highly effective method of gaining popularity is pet therapy. This subchapter explores the remarkable benefits of incorporating animal companionship into hospital settings and how it can positively affect the overall well-being of patients, their families, and even healthcare professionals.

The Healing Power of Pets:

Pets have an innate ability to provide comfort and unconditional love. Numerous scientific studies have shown that interacting with animals can reduce stress, anxiety, and depression while promoting relaxation and a sense of calm. In a hospital setting, where patients may be experiencing pain, fear, and isolation, the presence of a furry friend can work wonders by uplifting spirits and promoting emotional well-being.

Enhancing Physical Recovery:

It's not just health that receives help from pet therapy; physical recovery also improves. Studies say that petting or simply being in the presence of animals can lower blood pressure and heart rate, improve immune system function, and even reduce the need for pain medication. These physical benefits can accelerate healing and lead to shorter hospital stays, ultimately saving both patients and healthcare institutions time and money.

Creating a Positive Environment:

Pets have an uncanny ability to bring joy and laughter to any situation. By introducing therapy animals into hospitals, the atmosphere becomes more positive and uplifting. Patients and their families are provided with a welcome distraction from their worries and can focus on the joy and companionship these animals provide. This not only improves the overall experience for patients, but also for healthcare professionals, fostering a more positive work environment.

Complementing Traditional Treatments:

Pet therapy should not be considered a replacement for traditional medical treatments but rather as a complementary approach. The presence of animals can enhance the effectiveness of medical interventions, helping patients to better cope with their conditions, and promoting a faster recovery. By viewing pet therapy as an adjunct to conventional treatments, hospitals can offer a more integrated approach to patient care.

Incorporating pet therapy into hospital settings has the potential to unlock countless mental and physical health benefits for patients, families, and healthcare professionals alike. Whether it's a friendly dog, a gentle cat, or even a small therapy rabbit, the presence of these animals can alleviate stress, improve emotional well-being, and speed up physical recovery. By recognizing the power of pet companionship, hospitals can create a more compassionate and healing environment for all. After all, life is undeniably better when you have pets!

Chapter 6: Incorporating Pet Companionship into Self-Care

Establishing a Bond with Your Pet

Life is better when you have pets! The joy and companionship they bring into our lives are truly unparalleled. However, it is not enough to simply have a pet; it is equally important to prove a strong bond with them. In this subchapter, we will explore the several ways you can build a deep connection with your furry friend, enhancing the health benefits of pet companionship.

Primarily, communication is key. While our pets may not understand our words, they are incredibly perceptive to our tone of voice and body language. Take the time to speak to your pet in a gentle and reassuring manner. This will help them feel safe and loved, strengthening the bond between you. Additionally, be attentive to their needs and respond accordingly. Whether it is a scratch behind the ears or a treat for good behavior, positive reinforcement will reinforce the trust and affection they have for you.

Regular exercise and playtime are essential for both physical and emotional well-being. Engage in activities that your pet enjoys, such as playing fetch or going for a walk in the park. These shared experiences will strengthen the bond and provide an outlet for their energy and promote a healthy lifestyle for both of you.

Creating a routine is another effective way to show a bond with your pet. Animals thrive on structure and predictability. Set aside specific times for feeding, grooming, and play, allowing your pet to feel secure and comfortable in their environment. Consistency will help them understand expectations and foster a sense of stability and trust in your relationship.

Grooming is not only about keeping your pet's physical appearance but also a valuable opportunity to bond with them. Whether it is brushing their fur or trimming their nails, use these moments to show your pet love and care. It is a chance to relax together and build a stronger connection.

Lastly, always remember the power of touch. Physical contact, such as cuddling and petting, releases feel-good hormones for both you and your pet. These small gestures go a long way in reinforcing the bond and promoting a sense of security and comfort.

Ultimately, showing a bond with your pet is crucial for unlocking the health benefits of pet companionship. By communicating effectively, engaging in regular exercise and play, creating a routine, grooming, and embracing physical touch, you will deepen the connection with your furry friend. Life truly is better when you have pets, and with a strong bond, the joy and love they bring will enrich your life even more.

Creating a Pet-Friendly Environment

Pets bring immense joy and companionship to our lives, and it is important to create a pet-friendly environment that promotes their well-being and happiness. Whether you already have a furry friend or are considering getting one, understanding how to create a welcoming space for them is crucial. In this subchapter, we will explore various aspects of creating a pet-friendly environment and delve into the benefits it brings to both humans and their beloved animal companions.

First, it is essential to ensure the safety of your pet. Pet-proofing your home is a crucial step in creating a pet-friendly environment. This involves securing loose electrical cords, keeping toxic substances unreachable, and providing a designated space for them to rest and play. Investing in sturdy and safe pet-friendly furniture and removing any potential hazards will go a long way in preventing accidents and injuries.

Another key aspect of creating a pet-friendly environment is understanding their natural behaviors and needs. Providing many opportunities for exercise and mental stimulation is vital for their overall well-being. Designate areas in your home where they can play freely and consider incorporating interactive toys or puzzles to keep them engaged. Additionally, creating a routine for feeding, grooming, and playtime will help establish a sense of structure and security for both you and your pet.

Maintaining a clean and hygienic living space is equally important. Regularly cleaning their litter boxes, bedding, and toys will help prevent the spread of bacteria and ensure a healthy environment for everyone. It is also crucial to prove a pet-friendly outdoor space, such as a fenced-in yard or a designated walking area, where they can safely enjoy fresh air and exercise.

Lastly, a pet-friendly environment extends beyond just the physical aspects. It is essential to create an atmosphere of love, patience, and understanding. Spending quality time with your pet, showering them with affection, and providing positive reinforcement will strengthen the bond between you and your furry friend. Recognizing the unique needs and personalities of different pets will help you tailor your environment to suit them best.

As a result, creating a pet-friendly environment is a fundamental aspect of responsible pet ownership. By considering the safety, comfort, and well-being of our animal companions, we can unlock the countless health benefits that come with having pets. Remember, life is truly better when you have pets!

Pet Activities for Mental Well-being

Life is better when you have pets! There is no denying that the companionship of a furry friend can bring immense joy and happiness into our lives. But did you know that pets can also have a profound impact on our mental well-being? In this subchapter, we will explore the various pet activities that can unlock the health benefits of pet companionship.

1. Exercise and Outdoor Fun: Engaging in physical activities with your pet keeps them healthy and helps your well-being. Whether it's going for a walk, playing fetch in the park, or even hiking, these activities release

endorphins, reduce stress, and improve overall mood.

2. Mindful Moments: Take a moment to sit and observe your pet's behavior. Pay attention to their movements, their expressions, and the way they interact with their surroundings. This mindful observation can help you be present in the moment and bring a sense of calm and peace to your mind.

3. Pet-Assisted Therapy: Recently, pet-assisted therapy has gained recognition for its positive effects on health. Whether it's visiting hospitals, nursing homes, or participating in therapy sessions, the presence of animals can help reduce anxiety, lower blood pressure, and improve overall emotional well-being.

4. Creative Expression: Pets can be a great source of inspiration for creative activities. Take up painting, photography, or writing and capture the essence of your pet's unique personality. Engaging in these creative endeavors can provide a sense of fulfillment and act as a form of self-expression.

5. Bonding through Training: Training your pet helps in building a stronger bond and boosts your mental well-being. The process of teaching and learning new tricks stimulates your brain, improves cognitive abilities, and provides a sense of accomplishment.

6. Pet Meditation: Incorporating your pet into your meditation practice can deepen the experience. Find a quiet space, sit with your pet, and focus on their rhythmic breathing or the sensation of their fur

beneath your fingers. This practice can increase feelings of relaxation, reduce anxiety, and promote a sense of interconnectedness.

7. Emotional Support: Pets have an innate ability to sense our emotions and provide comfort during difficult times. Simply cuddling with your pet, sharing your thoughts, and receiving their unconditional love can have a significant positive impact on your mental well-being.

Remember, pets are not just companions, but also healers and teachers. By engaging in these pet activities, you can unlock the incredible health benefits that they offer. So, make time for your furry friends and let them be your guide on the path to improved mental well-being.

Chapter 7: The Science Behind Pet Therapy

Research Studies on Pet Therapy

Numerous research studies have been conducted to explore the benefits and effectiveness of pet therapy in improving health and overall well-being. These studies have provided compelling evidence that supports the notion that life is indeed better when you have pets! In this subchapter, we will delve into some of the most significant research findings on pet therapy.

One study conducted by the National Institute of Health found that interacting with animals, such as therapy dogs or cats, can significantly reduce stress levels. The presence of a friendly and non-judgmental animal companion helps to lower blood pressure, heart rate, and cortisol levels, which are commonly associated with stress. Pet therapy has also been found to increase the release of oxytocin, a hormone that promotes feelings of happiness and relaxation.

Another study published in the Journal of Psychiatric Research discovered that pet therapy can be particularly beneficial for individuals with health disorders, such as depression and anxiety. Participants who received regular pet therapy sessions reported a significant reduction in symptoms and an improvement in overall mood. The presence of animals has been shown to increase social interaction, decrease feelings of loneliness and isolation, and provide a sense of purpose and responsibility.

What's more, research conducted at universities and hospitals has highlighted the positive impact of pet therapy on specific populations, such as children with autism spectrum disorder (ASD) and elderly individuals with dementia. For children with ASD, interacting with therapy animals has been proven to enhance social skills, improve communication, and reduce disruptive behaviors. In the case of dementia patients, pet therapy has been found to alleviate agitation, increase engagement, and enhance quality of life.

The benefits of pet therapy extend beyond health. A study published in the Journal of the American Heart Association revealed that owning a pet, particularly a dog, is associated with a reduced risk of cardiovascular disease. Regular exercise with a pet, such as walking or playing, contributes to improved physical fitness and overall cardiovascular health.

All in all, numerous research studies have demonstrated the positive impact of pet therapy on health and overall well-being. Interacting with animals has been proven to reduce stress levels, alleviate symptoms of health disorders, enhance social interaction, and improve physical health. Therefore, it is evident that life is truly better when you have pets!

Theories Explaining the Benefits

There are numerous theories that attempt to explain the incredible health benefits that come from pet companionship. In this subchapter, we will delve into some of the most prominent theories to help you understand why life is undeniably better when you have pets!

One theory that has gained significant traction is the social support theory. Pets, especially dogs and cats, provide an unparalleled level of companionship and emotional support. They are always there for us, ready to lend an ear or simply provide a comforting presence. This unwavering loyalty and unconditional love can greatly reduce feelings of loneliness, anxiety, and depression. Having a pet by your side can create a sense of belonging and strengthen your social support network.

Another theory that explains the benefits of pet companionship is the biophilia hypothesis. This hypothesis suggests that humans have an innate desire to connect with nature and other living beings. Pets, being part of the natural world, fulfill this need by allowing us to establish a profound bond with another species. This connection with animals can promote feelings of calmness, relaxation, and overall well-being. It is no wonder that spending time with pets has been shown to reduce stress levels and improve mood.

The psychological theory of self-psychology also plays a role in understanding the benefits of pet companionship. Pets can serve as mirrors to our emotions, reflecting our feelings without judgment. This process allows us to better understand and regulate our emotions. In addition, caring for a pet can give us a sense of purpose and responsibility, fostering personal growth and self-esteem. Taking care of another living being can provide a sense of fulfillment and meaning in our lives.

The evolutionary theory suggests that humans have evolved to benefit from the companionship of animals. Throughout history, humans and animals have formed mutually beneficial relationships, with pets providing protection, hunting assistance, and emotional support. This theory explains why having a pet can tap into our evolutionary instincts and bring us a sense of contentment and happiness.

Everything considered, the numerous theories behind the health benefits of pet companionship provide us with a more profound understanding of why life is undeniably better when we have pets. Whether it is the social support they offer, the connection with nature they provide, the emotional reflection they offer, or even our evolutionary bond, pets bring immense joy and well-being into our lives. So, embrace the wonderful world of pet companionship and unlock the countless benefits that await you!

Understanding the Human-Animal Bond

Life is better when you have pets! For centuries, humans have formed deep connections with animals, and the bond between us and our furry companions is truly something special. In this subchapter, we delve into the fascinating world of the human-animal bond and explore the profound health benefits that come with pet companionship.

The human-animal bond refers to the unique and mutually beneficial relationship we share with animals. Whether it's a playful pup, a graceful feline, or even a small critter like a hamster or bird, pets have the incredible ability to bring joy, comfort, and a sense of purpose into our lives.

Research has shown that interacting with animals can have a positive impact on our mental well-being. When we cuddle with our pets, a hormone called oxytocin is released, promoting feelings of happiness and relaxation. This natural "love hormone" can help reduce stress, anxiety, and even alleviate symptoms of depression. What's more, the simple act of petting an animal can lower blood pressure and heart rate, resulting in a calmer state of mind.

Pets also provide companionship and a sense of belonging. They offer unconditional love and support, making us feel valued and needed. For individuals who may be struggling with feelings of loneliness or isolation, having a pet can be a lifeline, offering a constant source of comfort and companionship.

The responsibilities that come with pet ownership can have a positive impact on our health. Taking care of a pet provides structure and routine, giving us a sense of purpose and responsibility. This can be especially beneficial for individuals dealing with health issues, as it promotes a sense of self-worth and fosters a feeling of being needed and valued.

The human-animal bond is not limited to traditional pets like cats and dogs. Horses, for example, are often used in therapy programs known as equine-assisted therapy. These majestic creatures can help individuals struggling with trauma, anxiety, or other health conditions by providing a safe and non-judgmental environment for healing and personal growth.

In essence, the human-animal bond is a powerful force that enriches our lives in countless ways. Whether it's the joy of a wagging tail, the soothing purr of a cat, or the gentle nudge of a horse, pets have a remarkable ability to improve our mental well-being. So, embrace the love and companionship of a furry friend and experience the incredible health benefits that come with it. Remember, life is better when you have pets!

Chapter 8: The Future of Pet Therapy

Advancements in Animal-Assisted Interventions

Animal-assisted interventions have gained significant recognition in recent years as an effective therapeutic approach to improve health and overall well-being. This subchapter delves into the exciting advancements in this field, exploring how the power of pet companionship can truly transform lives. Whether you're a pet owner or considering bringing one into your life, understanding these advancements will reinforce the notion that "Life is better when you have pets!"

1. Canine-Assisted Therapy:

Canine-assisted therapy, also known as dog therapy, has emerged as a widely acclaimed animal-assisted intervention. Trained therapy dogs are now being deployed in various healthcare settings, including hospitals, nursing homes, and rehabilitation centers. These intelligent and loving animals offer emotional support, reduce anxiety, and even assist in physical rehabilitation. The latest advancements in this field have focused on specialized training programs for therapy dogs, enhancing their ability to respond to specific needs and conditions.

2. Feline-Assisted Therapy:

Cats, known for their calm and independent nature, are increasingly being recognized for their therapeutic potential. Feline-assisted therapy has been found to have a positive impact on individuals struggling with anxiety, depression, and even post-traumatic stress disorder. Recent advancements have focused on the development of structured interventions that utilize cats' unique qualities to create a soothing and nurturing environment. These interventions are proving to be particularly effective for individuals who may be more inclined towards cats than dogs.

3. Equine-Assisted Therapy:

Equine-assisted therapy, commonly known as horse therapy, has gained significant traction in recent years. Interacting with horses can be incredibly therapeutic, helping individuals develop self-awareness, communication skills, and emotional regulation. Advancements in this field have involved the integration of evidence-based practices, such as cognitive-behavioral therapy, alongside equine-assisted interventions. This combination ensures a holistic approach that addresses health challenges more comprehensively.

4. Exotic Animal-Assisted Therapy:

While dogs, cats, and horses are the most utilized animals in therapy, there has been a growing interest in the use of exotic animals. From dolphins to rabbits, these unique creatures offer distinct therapeutic benefits. Advancements in this area have focused on understanding the specific qualities of each exotic animal and tailoring interventions accordingly. This expansion of animal-assisted interventions allows for a wider range of options, ensuring that individuals can find the perfect furry or scaly companion for their therapeutic journey.

As we continue to unravel the health benefits of pet companionship, advancements in animal-assisted interventions offer new possibilities for improving the well-being of all humans. Whether it's the unwavering loyalty of a therapy dog, the calming presence of a therapy cat, the transformative power of interacting with horses, or the unique companionship of exotic animals, these advancements reinforce the belief that "Life is better when you have pets!" Embracing these advancements enhances our lives and recognizes the immense value that animals bring to our health and overall wellness.

Integrating Technology and Pet Companionship

In this digital age, technology has become an integral part of our lives, revolutionizing the way we communicate, work, and even relax. But did you know that technology can also enhance and enrich our relationships with our furry friends? Integrating technology and pet companionship can open a whole new world of possibilities for both humans and pets.

One of the most significant benefits of integrating technology with pet companionship is the ability to stay connected with your pet, even when you're away. With the help of smart devices and pet-specific apps, you can monitor your pet's activities, communicate with them, and even dispense treats remotely. This is particularly helpful for pet owners who have busy schedules or travel frequently, as it allows them to maintain a strong bond with their pets, even from a distance.

Another way technology can enhance pet companionship is through the wide range of interactive toys and games available. These innovative gadgets can provide mental stimulation for your pets, keeping them entertained and engaged when you're not available to play with them. From laser pointers to treat-dispensing puzzle toys, there's something for every pet's preference and personality. Not only does this help prevent boredom and destructive behavior, but it also strengthens the bond between you and your furry friend.

Technology can also assist in tracking and monitoring your pet's health and well-being. With the help of wearable devices like fitness trackers or GPS collars, you can keep tabs on your pet's activity levels, sleep patterns, and even locate them if they ever get lost. This not only ensures the overall well-being of your pet but also provides peace of mind for pet owners.

Additionally, integrating technology with pet companionship can open a whole new world of education and learning. Various apps and online platforms offer valuable resources on pet care, training techniques, and even virtual veterinary consultations. These technological tools can empower pet owners to make informed decisions about their pet's health and behavior, ultimately leading to better overall pet care.

As a result, integrating technology and pet companionship can provide numerous benefits for both humans and their beloved pets. From staying connected when apart, to providing mental stimulation and monitoring health, technology has the potential to enhance and enrich the bond between humans and their furry friends. Embracing these technological advancements can truly make the statement "Life is better when you have pets!" even more meaningful in today's digital world.

Expanding Access to Pet Therapy Programs

In recent years, there has been a growing recognition of the remarkable health benefits that come with pet companionship. From reducing stress and anxiety to improving overall well-being, pets have an incredible ability to provide comfort and support to humans. It is essential to expand access to pet therapy programs, allowing more individuals to reap the benefits of this unique form of therapy.

Pet therapy programs involve trained animals, typically dogs, who visit various settings such as hospitals, nursing homes, and schools to provide emotional support and companionship. These programs have proven to be incredibly effective in enhancing the health of individuals across all age groups. However, their availability and reach are limited, leaving many people unable to access this much-needed form of therapy.

Expanding access to pet therapy programs begins with increasing awareness and understanding of their benefits. It is crucial for individuals to recognize that pet companionship goes beyond mere companionship; it has the power to positively impact health. By educating the public about the benefits of pet therapy, we can encourage more organizations and institutions to incorporate these programs into their services.

Likewise, collaboration between healthcare providers, community organizations, and pet therapy programs is essential for expanding access. By working together, these stakeholders can develop innovative strategies to bring pet therapy programs to a wider audience. For instance, hospitals can establish partnerships with local pet therapy organizations to ensure that patients have regular interactions with therapy animals during their stay.

Additionally, financial support plays a crucial role in expanding access to pet therapy programs. Funding from both public and private sources can help cover the costs associated with training therapy animals, maintaining their health, and implementing programs in various settings. By advocating for increased funding and donations, we can ensure that pet therapy programs are accessible to individuals from all walks of life.

Ultimately, expanding access to pet therapy programs is a collective effort that requires the involvement of individuals, organizations, and communities. By recognizing the health benefits of pet companionship and working together, we can create a society where these programs are readily available to all who can benefit from them.

Remember, life is better when you have pets! By expanding access to pet therapy programs, we can unlock the incredible health benefits that come with pet companionship and improve the overall well-being of all humans. Let us join forces and make pet therapy programs accessible to everyone, ensuring a happier and healthier future for all.

Chapter 9: Ethical Considerations in Pet Therapy

Ensuring Animal Welfare

As humans, we have a responsibility to ensure the welfare and well-being of the animals that share our lives and our homes.

The bond between humans and animals is a special one, and it is our duty to provide them with the love, care, and respect they deserve. In this subchapter, we will explore the importance of ensuring animal welfare and how it contributes to the overall benefits of pet companionship.

One of the fundamental aspects of ensuring animal welfare is providing them with a safe and secure environment. Pets should have access to clean water, nutritious food, and appropriate shelter. Regular veterinary care is also essential to monitor their health and address any medical concerns promptly. By meeting these basic needs, we can ensure our pets live happy and healthy lives.

Physical exercise and mental stimulation are vital for the well-being of pets. Just like humans, pets require regular exercise to maintain a healthy weight and prevent obesity-related issues. Engaging in interactive playtime and providing them with toys and puzzles can keep their minds sharp and prevent boredom. Daily walks, runs, or play sessions benefit our pets and allow us to bond with them and stay active ourselves.

Another aspect of animal welfare is socialization. Pets are social creatures, and it is crucial to provide them with opportunities to interact with other animals and humans. Regular socialization helps prevent behavioral problems and ensures our pets are comfortable and confident in various situations. It is our responsibility to expose them to different environments, people, and animals, gradually and positively.

Responsible pet ownership also includes ensuring their safety. Microchipping, identification tags, and regular vaccinations are important measures to protect our pets from getting lost or falling ill. Additionally, spaying or neutering helps control the animal population and provides health benefits for our pets.

Lastly, it is crucial to treat animals with kindness and respect. They rely on us for their well-being, and it is critical to handle them gently, avoid physical punishment, and provide positive reinforcement for good behavior. By fostering an atmosphere of love and compassion, we create a strong bond with our pets and enhance their overall well-being.

It is crucial that ensuring animal welfare is an integral part of the benefits we gain from pet companionship. By meeting their basic needs, providing exercise and mental stimulation, promoting socialization, ensuring their safety, and treating them with kindness, we create an environment where both humans and animals thrive. Remember, life is better when you have pets, but it is our duty to ensure their happiness and well-being.

Training and Certification of Therapy Animals

In our quest to understand the numerous health benefits of pet companionship, we cannot overlook the significant role played by therapy animals. These remarkable creatures have been trained to provide comfort, support, and affection to individuals in need. Whether it's in hospitals, schools, or even disaster-stricken areas, therapy animals have proven time and again that their presence can make a world of difference. But how exactly are these animals trained and certified for such a crucial job?

Training therapy animals involves a combination of obedience training, socialization, and specific skill's development. Most therapy animals are dogs, but other animals, such as cats, horses, and rabbits, can also be trained for this purpose. The training process begins with basic obedience commands, such as sit, stay, and come. These commands ensure that therapy animals can be well-behaved and controlled in various settings.

Socialization plays a vital role in therapy animal training, as they must be comfortable interacting with people of all ages, backgrounds, and physical conditions. They are exposed to different environments, loud noises, and various stimuli to ensure they remain calm and unfazed during their therapy sessions. This process helps them adapt to different situations and personalities they may encounter during their work.

Additionally, therapy animals receive specialized training to perform specific tasks based on the needs of the individuals they will be assisting. For example, a therapy dog may be trained to perform tricks, retrieve objects, or even provide deep pressure therapy. These skills are tailored to meet the specific requirements of therapeutic settings, ensuring that the animals can provide maximum support to those in need.

Once the training is complete, therapy animals undergo certification processes to prove their suitability for therapy work. Certification typically involves an evaluation by a qualified professional who assesses the animal's behavior, obedience, and ability to handle different situations. This certification ensures that therapy animals meet specific standards of behavior, professionalism, and safety.

It is important to note that therapy animals should not be confused with service animals. While service animals are specifically trained to assist individuals with disabilities and have legal protections, therapy animals are trained to provide emotional support and companionship to a broader range of individuals without the same legal rights.

In brief, the training and certification of therapy animals are essential to ensure they can fulfill their roles effectively. Through obedience training, socialization, and specialized skill development, these animals become invaluable companions to individuals facing various health challenges. Their certification guarantees their ability to provide safe and reliable therapy to those in need. Therapy animals truly embody the sentiment that life is better when you have pets, as their presence brings comfort, joy, and healing to countless individuals.

Boundaries and Limitations in Pet Therapy

Pets have become more than just companions; they serve as valuable sources of support for our health. Pet therapy, also known as animal-assisted therapy (AAT), is a growing field that harnesses the power of the human-animal bond to improve overall well-being. However, it is essential to understand the boundaries and limitations involved in pet therapy to ensure the effectiveness and safety of this practice.

One crucial aspect of pet therapy is setting clear boundaries. While pets can provide immense comfort and emotional support, it is important to remember that they are not substitutes for human therapy or medication. Pet therapy should be considered a complementary approach rather than a standalone treatment. It is not meant to replace professional health care, but rather enhance it.

Another essential consideration is that not all pets are suitable for therapy purposes. Each animal has its temperament and personality traits that may or may not be suitable for engaging in therapy work. Not every pet is cut out for the demands and stresses of being a therapy animal. Therefore, it is crucial to carefully select animals that are well-trained, socialized, and comfortable interacting with strangers in various settings.

Additionally, it is essential to respect the boundaries of the animals themselves. Just like humans, animals have their own emotional and physical limits. Overworking therapy animals can lead to burnout, stress, and even behavioral issues. It is crucial to ensure that therapy animals are given ample rest, breaks, and downtime to recharge and maintain their well-being.

Plus, it is important to recognize that pet therapy may not be suitable for everyone. Some individuals may have allergies, phobias, or cultural beliefs that prevent them from fully benefiting from animal-assisted therapy. It is crucial to respect and accommodate these limitations while exploring alternative ways to support their health.

Lastly, it is important to note that pet therapy is not a one-size-fits-all solution. Different individuals may respond to different animals or species. While dogs are the most used therapy animals, other animals like cats, rabbits, horses, and even reptiles can also provide therapeutic benefits. It is essential to consider individual preferences and needs when selecting a therapy animal.

In summary, while pet therapy offers incredible health benefits, it is crucial to respect boundaries and limitations. Understanding that pets are not a substitute for professional treatment, selecting suitable therapy animals, acknowledging their limits, and recognizing individual preferences contribute to a successful and ethical pet therapy experience. By adhering to these boundaries, pet therapy can continue to enhance the lives of all humans, making life truly better when we have pets!

Chapter 10: Personal Stories of Transformation through Pet Companionship

Overcoming Health Challenges with a Pet

Life is better when you have pets! These furry companions not only bring joy and love into our lives but also offer a range of health benefits. In this subchapter of "Pets Make Better People: Unlocking the Health

Benefits of Pet Companionship," we explore the unbelievable ways pets can help us overcome health challenges. Whether you're struggling with anxiety, depression, or stress, your four-legged friend can be your greatest ally.

1. The Power of Unconditional Love:

Pets provide us with unconditional love, acceptance, and companionship. Their presence alone can instantly lift our spirits and make us feel valued. By having a pet by your side, you receive a constant reminder that you are never alone in your journey to overcome health challenges.

2. Stress Relief and Emotional Support:

Pets have a remarkable ability to alleviate stress and anxiety. They offer a sense of calm and stability, reducing the harmful effects of stress hormones in our bodies.

The simple act of stroking a pet's fur or playing with them releases endorphins, which promote feelings of happiness and relaxation.

3. Increased Social Interaction:

When battling health challenges, social isolation can often exacerbate our symptoms. Pets act as social facilitators, encouraging us to engage with others. Whether it's taking your dog for a walk or joining a pet-related community, pets create opportunities for social interaction, helping us build meaningful connections with fellow pet owners.

4. Routine and Responsibility:

Pets thrive on routine, and incorporating a pet into your life helps establish structure and responsibility. Having a set schedule for feeding, walking, and playing with your pet can provide a sense of purpose and stability, combating the unpredictability often associated with health challenges.

5. Sense of Purpose and Meaning:

Pets rely on us for their well-being, giving us a sense of purpose and meaning in life. When we care for a pet, we experience a boost in self-esteem and a renewed sense of responsibility. By nurturing our pets, we learn to nurture ourselves too, fostering personal growth and healing in the process.

Pets are not just furry companions; they are our allies in overcoming health challenges. Their unconditional love, stress-relieving abilities, social facilitation, routine, and sense of purpose all contribute to our overall well-being. So, if you're struggling with health issues, consider opening your heart and home to a pet. Discover the life-changing benefits of pet companionship and embark on a journey towards improved health and wellness. Remember, life truly is better when you have pets!

Finding Support and Healing in Unexpected Ways

Life is better when you have pets! They bring us joy, companionship, and a sense of purpose. But did you know that the benefits of pet companionship go far beyond the surface? In this subchapter, we will explore how our furry friends can offer us support and healing in unexpected ways.

Pets have an innate ability to sense our emotions and provide comfort when we need it the most. Whether you are feeling stressed, anxious, or lonely, your pet can be there for you in ways that humans sometimes can't. They offer us unconditional love and acceptance, creating a safe space for us to share our deepest thoughts and emotions without fear of judgment.

Often, we find healing in the simple act of caring for our pets. The responsibility of feeding, grooming, and exercising them encourages us to establish a routine and provides a sense of purpose. In return, our pets offer us a daily dose of laughter, playfulness, and affection. These interactions release endorphins, the feel-good hormones, which can help reduce stress and improve our overall well-being.

Again, pets can help us overcome emotional trauma and provide support during difficult times. They offer a non-judgmental presence, giving us the opportunity to express our pain and process our emotions in a safe environment. Their unconditional love and loyalty bring us a sense of security and stability, providing a much-needed anchor in times of crisis.

Additionally, pets can bridge the gap between humans, fostering social connections and reducing feelings of isolation. Taking our pets for walks or participating in pet-related activities can open doors to new friendships and communities. Sharing stories and experiences about our furry companions creates a common bond that can lead to lasting relationships and support networks.

Whether you are struggling with health issues, recovering from a loss, or simply searching for a source of comfort and companionship, pets can offer invaluable support. They have a unique ability to heal our wounds and bring us solace when we least expect it.

By and large, the benefits of pet companionship extend far beyond what meets the eye. Pets have an incredible capacity to provide support, healing, and a sense of belonging in unexpected ways. So, open your heart and let the paws of these remarkable creatures guide you towards a happier, healthier life. Remember, life truly is better when you have pets!

The Lifelong Impact of Pet Companionship

Pets have a profound impact on our lives, and their companionship can bring immeasurable joy, comfort, and wellness benefits. In this subchapter, we will delve into the lifelong impact of pet companionship and explore how having a furry friend can enhance our overall well-being. From childhood to old age, the presence of pets can greatly enrich our lives. Research has shown that growing up with pets can have a positive effect on a child's emotional and social development. Children who have pets tend to develop a sense of responsibility, empathy, and compassion. They learn about the cycle of life, develop better communication skills, and become more confident individuals. Pets also provide a constant source of unconditional love, helping children navigate through challenging times and providing a comforting presence during stressful situations.

As we transition into adulthood, the benefits of pet companionship continue to play a vital role in our lives. Pets offer companionship, reducing feelings of loneliness and providing a sense of purpose. They also encourage physical activity, as taking them for walks or playing with them promotes exercise and helps maintain a healthy lifestyle. The bond we form with our pets promotes stress reduction, lowers blood pressure, and decreases the risk of heart disease. Numerous studies have indicated that pet owners have lower levels of stress hormones and overall improved health compared to those without pets.

In the later stages of life, the presence of a pet can make a significant difference. Elderly individuals often experience feelings of isolation and depression, but having a pet can alleviate these emotions. Pets provide a sense of companionship, routine, and structure, which can contribute to a more fulfilling and active lifestyle. They offer unconditional love and emotional support, acting as a constant source of comfort during challenging times. On top of that, pets can help seniors stay mentally sharp by providing mental stimulation and a sense of purpose in their daily lives.

Putting it all together, pets have a lifelong impact on our well-being, bringing immense joy, comfort, and numerous health benefits. Whether we are children, adults, or seniors, the presence of a furry companion can enhance our emotional, social, and physical well-being. Life truly is better when we have pets, as they provide us with unwavering love, companionship, and a source of constant happiness.

Embracing the Healing Power of Pets

We often find ourselves searching for effective ways to improve our well-being. Look no further than the furry, four-legged companions that have been by our sides for centuries, our pets. Whether it's a loyal dog, a curious cat, a playful rabbit, or any other creature that captures our hearts, these animals offer more than just companionship; they hold the key to unlocking the health benefits that can enhance our lives.

Throughout this book, "Pets Make Better People: Unlocking the Health Benefits of Pet Companionship," we have explored the numerous ways in which pets improve our overall well-being. From the physical health benefits, such as reducing blood pressure and lowering the risk of heart disease, to the emotional support they provide during times of stress or grief, the healing power of pets is undeniable.

For all humans, life is undeniably better when you have pets. These incredible creatures offer us unconditional love, acceptance, and empathy. They are always there to greet us with wagging tails, purrs, or a gentle nudge, reminding us that we are loved and valued. Their presence alone has been shown to reduce feelings of loneliness and isolation, providing a sense of purpose and belonging.

Additionally, pets could bring joy and laughter into our lives. Their playful antics and amusing personalities can instantly lift our spirits and lighten our hearts. They encourage us to live in the present moment, reminding us to cherish the simple pleasures in life. Whether it's a game of fetch, a snuggle session on the couch, or watching them explore their surroundings with wide-eyed curiosity, our pets teach us the importance of finding joy in the little things.

In a world where we are constantly bombarded with stressors and demands, our pets offer us a respite from chaos. They provide a calming presence that can help alleviate anxiety and promote relaxation. The act of petting a dog or cat has been shown to release feel-good hormones such as oxytocin, serotonin, and dopamine, which can boost our mood and reduce stress levels.

So, whether you are a long-time pet owner or considering adding a furry friend to your family, remember the incredible healing power that pets possess. Embrace the love, joy, and support they bring into your life. Cherish the moments spent together, for they can improve your mental, emotional, and physical well-being. Life truly is better when you have pets!

Thank You for taking the time to read this eBook. I know first-hand the magical power of pets. I edited 4 motion pictures and wrote my first two published books with my two dogs and two cats all crowded in my studio. In their eyes you are their world, we cannot live without them.

Kevin